EFFECTIVE WAYS TO LOSE WEIGHT

102 TIPS ON FOODS AND EXERCISE TO LOSE WEIGHT

VICTOR AJAYI

EFFECTIVE WAYS TO LOSE WEIGHT: 102 TIPS ON FOODS AND EXERCISE TO LOSE WEIGHT

TABLE OF CONTENT

FORWARD

There was a time in our society when eating what mom cooked and going to work were the only options. The difference between that culture and ours is that people in the former worked on their feet in the fields or on a warehouse floor, not in front of a computer screen. The only way to work, and the reason it was termed work, was through physical labor. People could frequently eat everything they wanted during those times since they were burning off significantly more calories than they were taking in.

But like all things, that too has come to an end, and thanks to modern technology, we are now all overweight. Our comfort levels have grown tenfold, and our lives have changed so radically. Every rose has its thorn, as they say, and in our society, our desire for luxurious lifestyles and less work has started to show around the waistline.

The unfortunate aspect of it all is that the danger increases as your weight increases. If you don't do anything about it, illness—whether it takes the shape of diabetes or a heart condition—is guaranteed to manifest. It's not necessarily important to have a Built and Muscular body, but rather to be at a healthy weight. The abs can be worked on later; for now, you only need to lose a little additional body fat.

People are attempting to play catch up and operate from a position of weakness as society becomes aware of what is occurring and that we are overweight as a culture. They want to live a healthy lifestyle and shed some pounds.

We will help you lose the first 20 pounds with this eBook, which is something we all find difficult. It's remarkable how small lifestyle adjustments, which center around healthy diet and regular exercise, may help you drop 20 pounds.

CHAPTER 1

INTRODUCTION

Due to the fact that we are currently at an all-time high in our level of obesity, weight reduction and fat are such crucial aspects of our lives. Anybody listening in on a discussion or watching television will pay attention when the word "weight loss" is spoken. That's actually one of the most frequently searched keywords on the web right now.

Our relationship with food is the fundamental explanation of why we are so overweight. In our culture, we frequently place an emphasis on quantity. Instead of the best cuisine available, we simply want as much as we can obtain. When it should be the exact opposite, quantity always triumphs over quality.

It might be challenging to decide where to start once you've made the decision to reduce weight. It is achievable if you have a strong desire to start working out and lose weight. You simply need to learn how to say "ENOUGH IS ENOUGH".

Everyone is unique. Nobody one will have the same metabolism as you or burn fat in the same manner as you do. Even if you started an exercise and diet plan at the same time as the person next to you and followed the same routine every day, you Would not see the same results two weeks or even a month later.

Having said that, it's crucial to understand that not everyone uses food in the same way. What might make one individual gain a pound might not make another do the same. In order to lose weight, the same is true. Even if you eat and exercise exactly the same, you and your husband might not experience the same results if you're married and working out together. For example, if he stops drinking soda and loses five pounds as a result, but you don't, that proves that you and your husband are not the same.

The fact is that modern society has a lot more work to do than those in the past. Women and men were skinny sixty years ago because they had to work. You had to perform manual labor if you wanted to eat. If you wanted eggs, you had to go get them from the hen house. If you wanted fresh milk, you had to go milk the cows. And if you wanted to grow vegetables, you had to plow the fields. You had to be aware of the process of rearing a calf and having it killed if you desired beef. That was the way things were back then, but all of this laborious labor has been eliminated by technology. As a result, we must monitor our diet and force ourselves to exercise.

CHAPTER 2

EXERCISE IS BENEFICIAL FOR YOUR HEALTH

It just makes you feel nice all over when you recall a time when the sun and hard work were the causes of your sweat. You feel stronger all over as a result of the sun's direct impact on your shoulders and the tension it places on your muscles. Working out outside is the best thing there is.

The majority of people no longer work on farms, but a small number still get to experience the joy of doing work, creating something tangible, and maintaining a healthy weight while doing it. How many farm workers, cowboys, and ranchers are overweight, really? They are scarce. Consider their way of life. They get up, have breakfast and a cup of coffee, go to work, return for lunch, work, stay for dinner, and then go to bed early enough to get up the next morning and repeat the process. Meanwhile, they enjoy all-day access to fresh water, healthy exposure to the sun, and clean air. It really is a healthy way of living. Unfortunately, the majority of us spend our days sitting down inside working, while continuing to consume three meals per day, often without the chance to really enjoy them.

Except for those who live in cities where they can walk everywhere, it is a that city dwellers don't get much exercise. This implies that you must work hard and set your mind to it. You must incorporate exercise into your everyday routine to avoid being overweight and ill.

Exercise is the best approach to treat obesity, stress, hypertension, cardio vascular disease, and other disorders linked to a overweight lifestyle. It's better if you can workout outside, getting as much clean air as you can get is what your body needs.

CHAPTER 3

THE KEY IS CONSISTENCY

The most crucial component of any fitness plan is consistency. You can achieve your goals if you set them and continually work toward them. Most people find it simple to start. They go shopping, purchase some sport wear, running shoes, and perhaps a gym membership. After that, they engage in fairly consistent exercise for a week or two. However, they find it more difficult to stick to their fitness plan as they proceed. Their daily obligations increase, and they start going to the gym less frequently. In other words, they simply quit attending to the gym after their subscription is wasted.

Even though many people prefer to exercise in the evenings, other people find it more difficult to stick with this schedule. This is an excellent time to exercise if you are not entirely worn out from work. However, if you are unable to, you might need to do it in the morning.

Contrary to popular belief, exercise doesn't always leave you feeling exhausted. It might affect you in this way at first, but as you get fitter, you'll notice that you have more energy. You shouldn't have any trouble getting up in the morning and getting going if you combine exercise with enough sleep. Additionally, you'll be energized the entire day, which will make it lot simpler for you to get through your job.

Even if you don't belong to a gym, there's a good possibility that your home has a sidewalk, and some people might even have access to a pool. Get up 30 minutes early, put on your sneakers, and start walking, running, jogging, or doing whatever activity you want. Your four-legged companion will undoubtedly enjoy spending time with you as well.

CHAPTER 4

FOODS

People overlook the fact that cutting the first 20 pounds involves changing what they eat.

Below are tips about food to follow to help you reduce weight.

No 1: Limit your intake of coffee as it can make your body less sensitive to the natural fat-burning properties of caffeine. maximum of one or two glasses (if the day starts out fairly slowly).

No 2: Try to drink your tea and coffee black if you must have them. Black tea or coffee can be beneficial to your health as long as you drink plenty of water to balance the caffeine in them. Caffeine is also bad for you since it interferes with bodily processes like metabolism.

No 3: Green tea is another variety of tea that you are free to consume. Over 4,000 years ago, green tea was utilized as medicinal in China. It supports the digestive system, can ease an excessively full stomach, and has been connected to a lower chance of developing cancer.

No 4: Don't worry about cheating, but avoid doing so during meals. Consume treats and your favorite cheat food solely for flavor. Share a dessert with the entire family if you desire one after dinner. You won't gain any weight, just the flavor.

No 5: While white bread is good, multigrain breads strong in fiber are considerably superior. These breads provide a good amount of protein and are an additional approach to increase your diet's fiber intake.

No 6: Avoid foods with no or low fat content. These food products are widely available, although they are not particularly healthful. Many of these foods are sweetened with a chemical or carbohydrate to improve their flavor. These substances and carbohydrates are nevertheless converted by the body into sugar, which implies that fat is still formed from them.

No 7: Fats should make up 15-20% of your meal. This is really all the fat your body needs. A lot of this is going to be in your diet in the form of cream, sugar and the like.

No 8: Fresh vegetables are preferable to canned ones, just like fruits. If you can eat your vegetables raw, that is even better. The nutrients are lost when you cook them. If you must cook them, try to boil them just long enough to keep some of their crispness. Don't dunk them in butter either. It would be best if you could purchase organic vegetables free of pesticides..

No 9: Be mindful of everything you eat, from the dish itself to the garnishes. A healthy dinner might be ruined by garnishes and condiments because they frequently include a lot of fat.

No 10: Only 25–30% of your diet should be made up of proteins. The idea that meat should be the focal point of your meal is overemphasized. In reality, it is more appropriate to classify it as a side dish as opposed to the main meal.

No 11: It is preferable if you can refuse alcohol. Although a glass of red wine is good for heart, most alcoholic beverages are just fattening. Particularly fattening is beer. Depending on the ingredients they include, cocktails can make you fat. Take whiskey with Coke as an example. The Coke is undoubtedly fatty, but the whiskey might not be. Additionally, most people get drunk after a few drinks, and when you're a little tipsy and hungry, you won't be able to make sane decisions about your diet. It's also common to overeat in the late evening, right before you pass out from a night of drinking. Simply put, the entire mix is poor.

 No 12: Try to have breakfast an hour after waking up. The greatest method to give your body the boost it needs is to do this. Avoid waiting till you are genuinely hungry. Although breakfast is crucial, you shouldn't overeat. You're supposed to be breaking your fast after not eating all night.

No 13: Work off the extra calories by the end of the week. Make sure to visit the gym or go for a longer walk if you feel like you have indulged excessively this week in order to burn off those additional calories.

No 14: Try to avoid soda as much as possible. All sodas are heavily sugar sweetened. It's best to eliminate as much of your diet as you can. Diet soda is still soda, too. Despite having less sugar, it still contains additional chemicals and ingredients that are bad for your health. When consuming soda, follow it up with a glass of water. Keep in mind that caffeine also dehydrates you. Sodas that have been decaffeinated still include small levels of caffeine and the same amount of sugar, making them not significantly healthier.

No 15: Have a glass of water before you start eating. Drinking water will help you feel fuller naturally, reducing the amount of food you need to eat.

No 16: Use less salt overall and make an effort to reduce it in half. One of the biggest contributors to obesity is salt.

No 17: Try to cut back on your sugar intake. If you must sweeten your coffee and tea, look for an artificial sweetener whose flavor you enjoy. However, these activities should also be restricted because they are not particularly healthy either.

No 18: Vegetables make excellent snacks. If you are experiencing hunger pangs, they can help you get through them, because they are nutrient-rich and satiate hunger, carrots are wonderful.

No 19: Try to avoid snacking in between meals, but if you must, make sure it's a healthy snack. Try to find healthy snacks rather than junk food if you travel frequently..

No 20: Don't drink too much tea or coffee. If you don't add a lot of cream and sugar to them, they are essentially safe. The cream and sugar turn into fatty ingredients. Consider it this way, every time you drink a cup of coffee or tea with cream and two sugar cubes, it's like eating a piece of chocolate cake. Imagine how much cake you will consume after drinking a Venti Starbucks Latte; ouch.

No 21: Eating pork in no way promotes weight loss. You will do better when trying to lose weight if you consume less pork. Bacon, ham, and sausage are among the foods made from pork, which has a high fat content.

No 22: Try dry wine if you must consume alcohol. Due to the higher sugar content in sweet wines, dry wine is preferable. Although dry wines include sugar, the majority of it has been fermented into alcohol, making them better.

No 23: Include foods from each food group in your daily diet. This is a fantastic technique to make sure you are getting all the nutrients your body need and it aids in preventing any dietary deficits. Additionally, avoid eating the same things repeatedly. Try new things to avoid getting bored with your diet..

No 24: Only eat if you are truly hungry. First take sips of some water to ascertain whether you are hungry or just really thirsty. It's common for people to eat when they see food. They simply want to consume it; it does not imply that they are hungry. If you're not truly hungry, don't accept any food that is offered to you. If you feel obligated to eat it out of politeness, simply nibble; skip a meal.

No 25: Drink a glass of clean, fresh water to start your day. Drink one as soon as you awaken in the morning. Because your body won't be resisting, it will be easier for it to start.

No 26: Control your sweet tooth. You can still enjoy your favorite sweets as long as you don't consume them as a meal. Always keep in mind that these treats contribute to a situation that you don't want them to contribute to. However, don't deprive yourself either because you'll eat twice as much as you ought to.

No 27: Choose fresh fruit over fruit that has been processed, or anything that is converted into additional sugar. Fruits that have been processed or canned likewise lack the fiber that fresh fruits possess.

No 28: Avoid being a victim of crash diets. These are detrimental to your health and ultimately cause more harm than good. Usually, you will drop a few pounds in the short term, but as soon as you stop, everything returns, making your weight worse than before. You ultimately reach a point where you must stop following a crash diet because you cannot thrive on one.

No 29: Watch your fat intake. A gram of fat contains 9 calories. You can calculate the quantity of fat in those things if you know your overall calorie intake.

No 30: Eat more white meat than red meat. Chicken, fish, and some other poultry are examples of white flesh. Beef and pork are examples of red meat.

No 31: If you're attempting to reduce weight, vegetables are your buddies. You might even want to try some of the options that you haven't tried before because there are so many to choose from. Leafy greens are the best kind of vegetables, so whenever you can, include salads in your meals. Salads are nutrient-dense as long as you don't overdress them or pile on too many toppings.

No 32: Water is wonderful. Over 66% of your body weight is made up entirely of water. For the same reason, water is crucial for keeping a healthy weight.

Drink plenty of water. Even though it may take you some time to get there, the recommended daily intake is eight glasses. Water is essential for your body. Water not only helps your body eliminate waste, but it also lifts your spirits and Water not only cleanses your body of toxins but also enhances your health and happiness. When you drink a lot of water, you just start to feel fit, and this gives you the motivation to lose weight. Water contains no calories, so you can consume as much as you wish without feeling guilty. You will eat less if you drink a lot of water since you won't feel like you're starving to death. Never forget that if you feel hungry, you were most likely only thirsty and not at all hungry.

No 33: You should aim to drink the recommended eight glasses every day. The simplest way to do this and track your water intake is to get a jug from a drugstore or grocery store that is designed to hold exactly 8 glasses of water. Since you can fill them up, freeze them, and then drink fresh, cold water all day as the ice melts, these are wonderful weight-loss tools. If you don't mind, you can also drink your water at room temperature. It just matters that you are consuming the necessary amounts of water for your body.

No 34: Don't believe what you hear about fruit juice being healthy. In actuality, juice contains a sizable amount of sugar. If you're in the mood for a glass of juice, opt for fresh fruit juice rather than juice with added flavors and colors. Making your own fruit juice is even preferable. Be careful not to add too much sugar as that will increase the calories. Eat more fruit instead of drinking fruit juice.

Fruit supplies your body with essential fiber and vitamins.

No 35: Use high-quality extra virgin olive oil while cooking using oil. It is more expensive than vegetable oil, but because of the superior health advantages, the price is justified. Olive oil helps to increase the elasticity of the arterial walls, which lowers the risk of heart attack and stroke. It has also been linked to a lower risk of coronary heart disease.

No 36: Whether it's liquid meals, desserts, or ice cream, chew it at least 8 to 12 times. Saliva is added to the food, aiding in the sugar's digestion. When food isn't thoroughly chewed and is instead just swallowed, you flood your stomach with indigestible food that doesn't provide the necessary health advantages.

No 37: Drink some water along with your meal. Drink something after every bite to help you

feel filled without feeling bloated and to help you finish your meal more quickly. Drinking water while you eat will also help your meal to settle more quickly, which also helps you to feel full faster.

No 38: Use non-stick frying pan spray to avoid using oil. Additionally, non-stick pans require little to no oil at all.

No 39: Avoid eating anything that has been fried. If it is breaded, baking it is preferable. Foods that are fried are covered in fat and oil. Even after the extra oil has been removed, oil is still absorbed into the food item.

No 40: Don't skip meals. A minimum of three meals each day are recommended, but five small meals are preferred. As a result, you won't become ravenous during the day and end up overeating.

No 41: Instead of frying or roasting veggies, boil them, but not for too long. You can also steam them, which is likely the healthiest way to consume foods like carrots, broccoli, cauliflower, and cabbage.

No 42: Consume water-rich fresh produce like fruits and vegetables. These include items such as tomatoes, watermelons, cantaloupe, kiwi, grapes, etc. All of those luscious, fresh fruits and vegetables are healthy for you. Since these foods are between 90 and 95 percent water, you can eat a lot of them and they won't make you gain weight.

No 43: Increase your intake of fiber as much as you can. Typically, this entails consuming more fruits and vegetables..

No 44: Limit your egg consumption to one per day. The ideal scenario is to limit your weekly egg consumption to three.

No 45: Try to eat as many vegetarian meals as you can. Even if you can't entirely cut out meat, this is still a better way of living. It is better to consume as many fruits and vegetables as you can. The more meat you eliminate from your diet, the more fat you may eliminate as well. However, protein is crucial, so be sure your choice enables you to maintain healthy protein levels.

No 46: Your diet should include all aspects of the food groups including carbohydrates. In fact, your diet needs to be about 50-55% carbs. Carbs are a great source of energy. Those diets that prohibit carbohydrates are actually harming you and only making you crave them that much more. Your diet should not cause you to be deficient in anything.

No 47: Chocolates should be treated as luxury items. Buy the good stuff and only eat them every once in awhile. If you really savor each morsel, you'll experience that much more joy in eating them and they will taste even better.

No 48: Set a time for meals and stick to it. Try to schedule your meals so that you can consume them at those times. You can manage when and what you eat by developing an eating routine. Additionally, eating five little meals throughout the day is preferable to just one or two large ones. Your body feels as though it is famished when you only eat once a day, which causes it to store fat rather than use it as fuel. Do not wait until you are famished before eating. You will only eat excessively till full as a result of this.

No 49: Avoid impulse Eat, eat only when you are hungry.

CHAPTER 5

EXERCISE

To start improving and getting your body into shape, it takes longer than a week. Many people make the error of thinking that their exercise is ineffective when it only requires a brief period of time.

If you push your body too much when you first get started exercising you can end up with injuries. Your ligaments, joints, and bones are not designed to withstand the strain you are placing on them. Do not believe that if you really push yourself during a few workouts that you will lose fat; sadly, this is not how the body functions. Slow and steady wins the race..

Below are some workout tips to follow

No 1: You can get your daily 10 minutes of cardio through activities other than running..

No 2: Don't let the fact that your clothes don't fit stop you from working out and eating healthy. Wear a medium if you are that size. The improper kinds of clothing can give you the impression that you are bigger than you actually are. This also applies to athletic wears. If you wear clothing that fits today, you can shop later for smaller clothing.

No 3: Stand up and stretch every 30 minutes or so if you work a job that requires you to sit for the entire shift. The majority of today's occupations demand you to sit down in front of a computer. Make it a point to move occasionally if you have a job like this.

No 4: Take a rest when your body signals that it has had enough. You will begin to receive messages from your body once you have exercised for a while. When you are just beginning your fitness plan, it's crucial to adhere to such signals.

No 5: Don't slump in your chair. At all times, try to sit up straight and erect. Slouching makes you seem flabby and is unhealthy for your back. Make it a point to maintain proper posture while standing and sitting.

No 6: Always begin and conclude your workout with a 5–10 minute warm-up and 5–10 minute cool-down, respectively. Before responding well to the remainder of the workout, your body must attain a certain heart rate threshold.

No 7: To tone your midsection, use pelvic gyrations. These are obviously not exercises you would perform in public, but they are a fantastic first step in getting your body ready for more challenging stomach crunches. It keeps you loose rather than tight and is also helpful for your back muscles.

No 8: If you can sit, do not lie down.

No 9: Take a walk with your dog. If you're not exercising enough, there's a good chance your pet isn't either. Alternately, let your dog walk you. Allow him to lead you for once in his life in the direction and at the pace he chooses. Both of you might benefit from the workout.

No 10: Walking around while on the phone. If the chat is lengthy, you'll get a nice workout.

No 11: Don't let your cell phone or smartphone be close by. Walk to it if it rings. Life is full with conveniences, and everything we need is always nearby, yet this is obviously detrimental for our health.

No 12: Gradually lengthen your workouts if you chose to do so. The same is true of your workout intensity.

No 13: Instead of going up the stairs one at a time, go up them twice. Your heart rate goes up as a result of having to push yourself more.

 No 14: Gather knowledge on exercises and simple tasks you may complete at home. There is a ton of in-depth research on exercise accessible, and you may chose what will help you the most to achieve your weight loss objectives. For further information on how to burn the target number of calories you want to burn each week, browse the web or have a look at some books on health and fitness that you can find at your local library or bookstore..

No 15: Move around instead of remaining still. Do it if you can move around. Pacers actually benefit greatly from their frequent movement since it helps them stay healthy. You can think better through pacing.

No 16: Do things yourself. Walk and get it yourself if you need something from the kitchen, the TV station changed, the mail, or the newspaper from the driveway. You'll benefit greatly from including some walking in your daily routine.

No 17: Take a day off from working out to give your body a chance to recover and mend.

Every week, your body requires a day off.

No 18: Before going to bed, take off your clothes and examine yourself in the mirror. Make a list of the things you need to work on and the things you do best. Making a self-inventory might help you stay inspired as you work out. Don't forget to congratulate yourself on any new muscle tone or other changes you may have achieved.

No 19: If you're on the bus or train, get off a few blocks before your stop and continue walking from there. This is a convenient method to get in a walk before and after work or when going to somewhere else.

No 20: Move around or perform easy workouts like crunches or leaning over and touching your toes during breaks. Do whatever it takes to keep your blood circulating and your body moving.

No 21: Look for a workout partner. This person should share your commitment to exercise and weight loss. Finding a devoted partner has several benefits, one of which is having someone to feel accountable to. It is simpler to get out of bed and go for a workout with someone when you know they are waiting for you. You wouldn't want to stand up your workout partner, would you?

No 22: Play some music and get up and move. It goes without saying that the more you move, the better you'll feel and the more weight you'll shed.

No 23: People underestimate the amount of fat that muscle training can burn. When you work on developing muscle, your body starts to burn fat as fuel for your growing muscles. Be aware that because muscle weighs more than fat, your scale might not accurately reflect your weight loss as you add muscle.

No 24: If you can stand, avoid sitting. You can burn more calories by standing than by sitting if you can do so comfortably.

No 25: When you walk, breathe through your nose. Maintain a normal gait while making an effort to tuck your stomach in. Soon, you'll start to feel those muscles tighten.

No 26: Join a dancing class. This can involve learning ballroom dances like the fox trot, salsa, or tango. Those fast-moving dances will have you moving. Ballroom dancing is a vigorous workout and will tone your legs even when done slowly.

Alternately, enroll in an aerobic dancing class. How many overweight dancers are you familiar with?

No 27: Pick a workout plan that works for your lifestyle. Everyone has a distinct lifestyle and works in a different field. There is no specific time that you must or must not exercise. If you find that working out late before bed is calming for you, then do it. It's also fantastic if you prefer to exercise first thing in the morning because it helps you wake up. Due to the stress of their jobs or because it is the only time they have available, some people like working out during their lunch break.

No 28: If you have the time, walk everywhere. Consider walking or riding a bicycle if the distance to work or the grocery store is short. While it might take a little longer, you'll still be working out.

No 29: The majority of people want to target and completely eliminate their stomachs. We're unable to spot reduce, unfortunately. However, one thing you can do to assist tone your stomach muscles is to practice deep breathing, tuck your stomach in as much as you can while inhaling as forcefully as you can. Hold it for a few seconds before releasing it gradually. Avoid letting it out so quickly that you flip over. Not good at all. When you think about it, try to breathe in this way; 50–60 times a day is optimal. This will assist you in losing at least an inch in around 20 days.

No 39: Give up smoking. Although smoking may not directly affect your weight, it does cause unpredictable eating patterns and increases caffeine dependence.

No 40: Practice breathing techniques to trim your middle. It is incredible how properly breathing and using your entire diaphragm may actually aid in toning your abs. The majority of individuals already breathe far too little, which is bad for the brain since it requires enough oxygen.

No 40: You can maintain your weight with three days of 30 minutes of exercise, but to start losing weight, you need at least four days of 30 minutes of activity, and five days a week is even better.

When you begin exercising, weigh yourself, but don't take the results as a gauge for how much weight you are losing. Your weight changes during the course of the day. If you weigh yourself every day, you might simply end up giving up.

No 41: Use the stairs rather than the escalator or elevator. Despite being wonderful conveniences, these things make us exceedingly lazy. Additionally, taking the stairs can be quicker than waiting for an elevator to open.

No 42: Try 15 minutes of brisk walking to stay in shape if you are unable to run due to a physical condition.

No 43: You can either take the stairs or the escalator to keep up with it.

No 44: The couch and the TV are detrimental to losing weight. Avoid sitting on it if you have a tendency to become a couch potato. In order to reduce the amount of time you spend in front of the television, if necessary, place a less comfortable chair in front of it. In the case of computer junkies, the same holds true. Some individuals find their chairs to be more comfortable in front of their computers than in front of their televisions. (Of course, if you don't work from home and must spend hours at a time sitting in front of a computer, your chair is crucial.)

No 45: Swim every time you can. Swimming is a wonderful cardio workout that has little to no pressure on the joints, making it ideal for those with osteoporosis or other joint issues.

No 46: Try playing basketball or tennis. Playing video games is a terrific way to exercise. In a competitive setting, working out with a partner is also more enjoyable. Just be careful not to overdo it. You'll be more motivated to push yourself and burn more calories.

No 47: If you're standing about, try standing on your toes for a moment before lowering yourself to your heels to stretch your legs out a bit. You can also flex your buttocks, but perhaps only if no one else is around.

No 48: Push your body away from the wall with your hands while leaning against it with your face near to it. Stretch by repeating this three or four times.

No 49: Reward yourself when you frequently check your weight and the way your clothes fit. Purchase a new pair of pants or a new pair of running shoes for yourself. As you work toward your weight loss objectives, this will support you in staying motivated.

No 50: Keep the remote out of sight. Additionally harmful to weight loss are remote controllers. Without a remote, you might not even turn on the TV, which means you might look for more engaging activities to do. If you don't have a remote, get up and change the station, or go for a walk in place of watching TV.

No 51: Give yoga a try. Yoga is a fantastic method to get in shape and relieve tension. Through yoga, you can learn to manage your muscles and increase the control you have over each specific muscle group.

No 52: The best indicator that you are losing weight is how well your clothes fit. You'll know that eating right and exercise are helping you if you start to feel like you're floating around in your clothes. Moving where you normally fasten your belt—tighter is obviously better—is another sign that you're losing weight.

No 53: Don't give up if you don't notice results immediately when you start working out, whether at home or in a gym.

9 7 9 8 8 4 8 7 1 8 4 9 2